Resources for Further Learning and Support

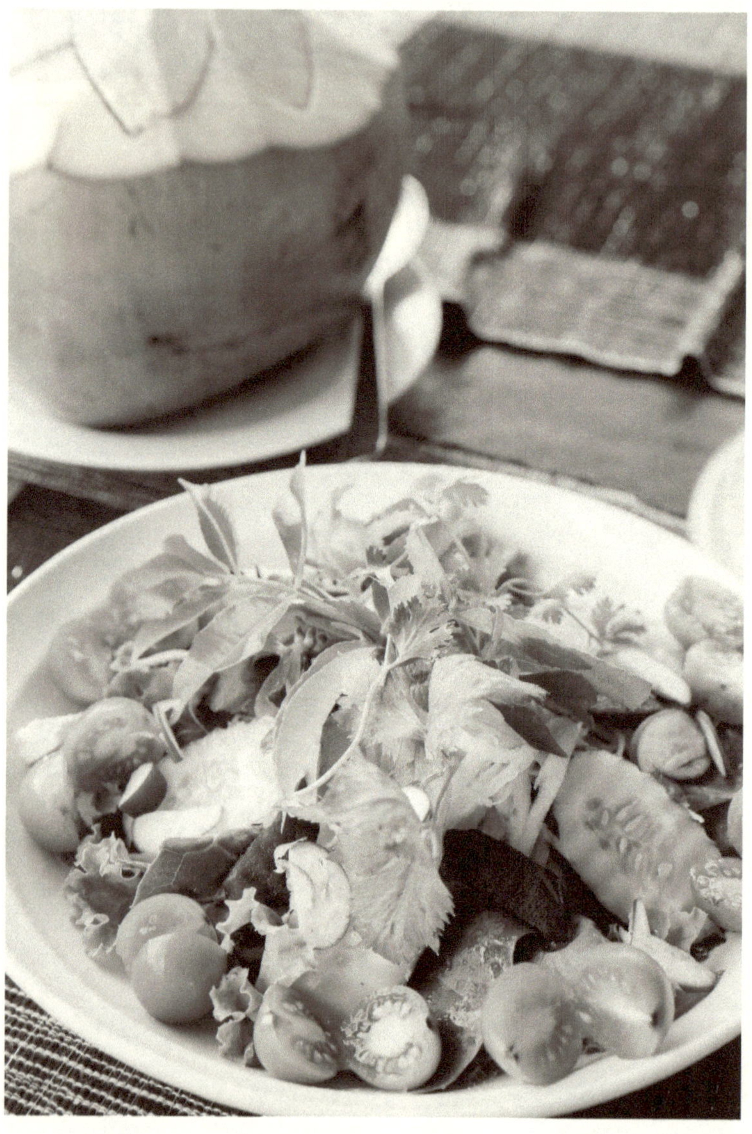

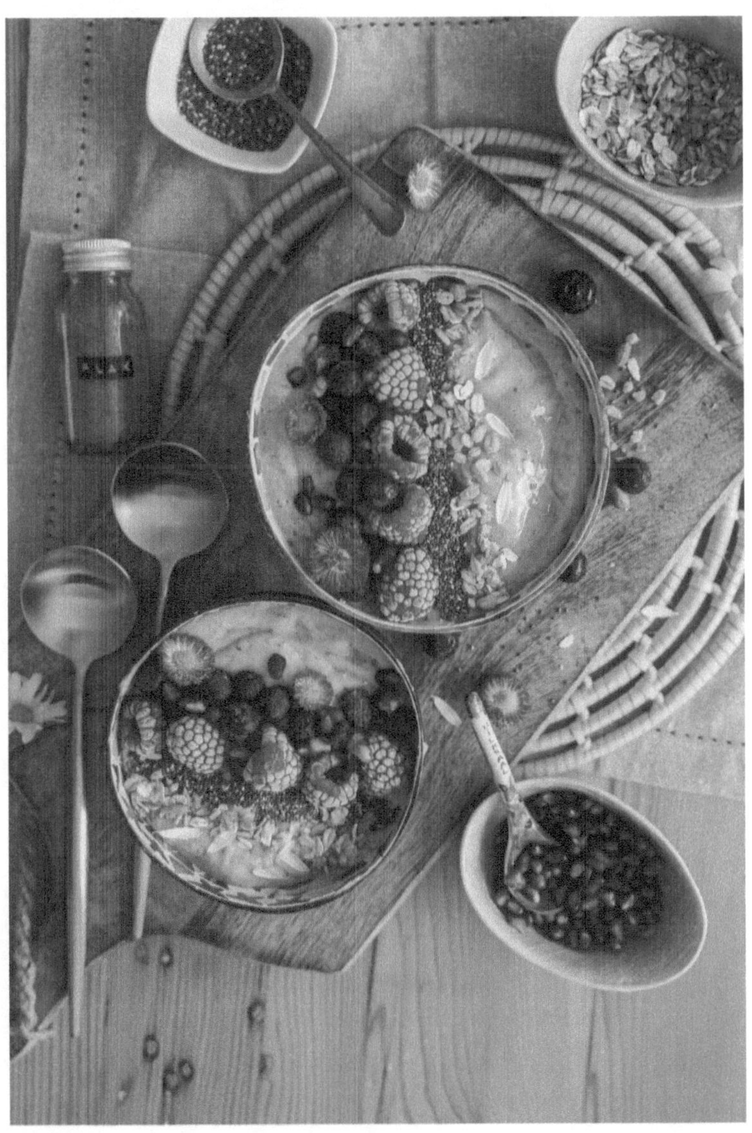

Chapter 1: The Basics of Vegan and Plant-Based Cooking

Are you interested in trying a vegan or plant-based diet, but aren't sure where to start when it comes to cooking? Don't worry, you're not alone. Transitioning to a vegan or plant-based diet can seem overwhelming at first, but with the right guidance, it can be a rewarding and delicious lifestyle choice.

In this chapter, we'll cover the key ingredients and techniques that form the foundation of vegan and plant-based cooking. Whether you're new to the kitchen or an experienced cook looking to try something new, we'll help you feel confident and prepared to create delicious, plant-based meals.

Let's start with the basics. What exactly is a vegan or plant-based diet? At its core, a vegan diet excludes all animal products, including meat, dairy, eggs, and even honey. A plant-based diet, on the other hand, centers around whole, minimally processed foods that come from plants, including fruits, vegetables, whole grains, legumes, nuts, and seeds. While these two diets share many similarities, it's important to note that not all vegan foods are necessarily healthy, and not all plant-based foods are necessarily vegan.

So, where do you start when it comes to cooking vegan and plant-based meals? Here are a few key ingredients to add to your pantry:

Legumes: Beans, lentils, and chickpeas are versatile sources of protein that can be used in soups, stews, salads, and more.

Whole Grains: Brown rice, quinoa, and oats are filling and nutrient-dense, and can be used as a base for many different meals.

Nutritional Yeast: This flaky, cheesy-tasting seasoning is a staple in vegan cooking, and can be used to add flavor to soups, sauces, and more.

Nuts and Seeds: Almonds, cashews, sunflower seeds, and pumpkin seeds can be used to make vegan cheese, sauces, and dressings.

Plant-Based Milks: Soy, almond, and oat milk are all great alternatives to dairy milk, and can be used in recipes or as a standalone beverage.

Now that you have a few key ingredients on hand, it's time to get familiar with some basic cooking techniques. Here are a few that you'll use frequently in vegan and plant-based cooking:

Sautéing: This involves cooking food in a small amount of oil or liquid over high heat. It's great for cooking veggies, tofu, and tempeh.

Roasting: Roasting vegetables in the oven is a great way to bring out their natural sweetness and add depth of flavor. Try roasting broccoli, cauliflower, or sweet potatoes.

Boiling: This is a simple and fast way to cook grains and legumes. Simply add them to boiling water, and let them cook until tender.

Blending: A high-speed blender is a great tool for making smoothies, sauces, and soups.

Baking: Vegan baking involves substituting ingredients like eggs, butter, and milk with vegan alternatives. You can still make delicious cookies, cakes, and breads without animal products!

With these key ingredients and techniques in your arsenal, you're ready to start experimenting with vegan and plant-based cooking. Don't be afraid to try new things and get creative in the kitchen. Who knows, you might just discover a new favorite dish!

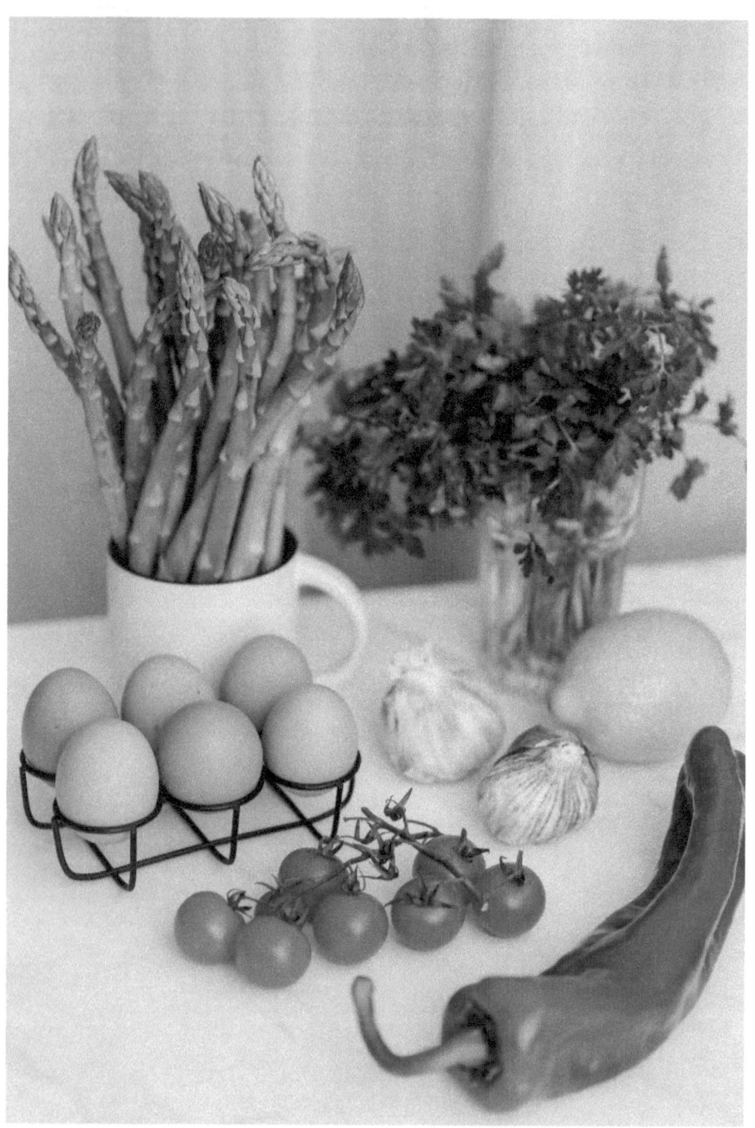

Chapter 2: Plant-Based

Proteins - Ditching Meat and Finding Complete Proteins in a Vegan Diet

Protein is essential for maintaining a healthy body and a balanced diet. However, many people think that a vegan or plant-based diet is not capable of providing enough protein to meet their needs. Fortunately, this is a myth - a well-planned vegan diet can easily provide all the necessary protein, without relying on animal products. In fact, many plant-based sources of protein are healthier than their animal counterparts.

One of the biggest misconceptions about plant-based protein is that it is incomplete, meaning it does not contain all nine essential amino acids that our body needs to function properly. While it is true that some plant-based sources of protein are incomplete, there are plenty of options that are complete proteins, containing all the essential amino acids. Examples include soy products like tofu and tempeh, quinoa, chia seeds, hemp seeds, and seitan.

Soy products, including tofu and tempeh, are excellent sources of complete protein, with 10-20 grams of protein per serving. Tofu is a versatile ingredient that can be used in savory and sweet dishes, while tempeh has a nutty flavor and a firmer texture that works well in sandwiches, stir-fries, and salads.

Quinoa is a seed that is often considered a grain due to its texture and cooking properties. It is also a complete protein, with 8 grams of protein per cup of cooked quinoa. Quinoa is a versatile ingredient that can be used in salads, stir-fries, soups, and as a base for grain bowls.

Chia seeds and hemp seeds are two more complete protein sources that are also rich in healthy fats and fiber. Chia seeds can be used to make a delicious pudding, while hemp seeds are great for adding to smoothies and salads.

Seitan is a protein-rich food made from wheat gluten. It has a meaty texture that makes it a popular meat substitute in vegan cooking. Seitan can be grilled, baked, fried, or used in stews and casseroles. It has around 25 grams of protein per 3-ounce serving.

It is important to note that while these plant-based sources of protein are complete proteins, it is not necessary to consume them in one meal or even one day. Our body stores amino acids and can use them as needed, so as long as we are eating a varied diet throughout the day and week, we are likely getting all the essential amino acids we need.

In addition to the complete proteins, there are plenty of incomplete protein sources that can be combined to make a complete protein. Some examples include beans and rice, peanut butter on whole grain bread, and hummus with pita bread.

If you are concerned about getting enough protein on a vegan diet, it can be helpful to track your protein intake using a food diary or an app like MyFitnessPal. The recommended daily intake of protein is about 0.8 grams per kilogram of body weight, so for a 150-pound person, that would be about 55 grams of protein per day.

In conclusion, plant-based sources of protein are abundant and easy to find. Incorporating a variety of plant-based protein sources into your diet can provide all the essential amino acids your body needs. By ditching meat and incorporating more plant-based protein into your diet, you can reap the benefits of a healthier and more sustainable lifestyle.

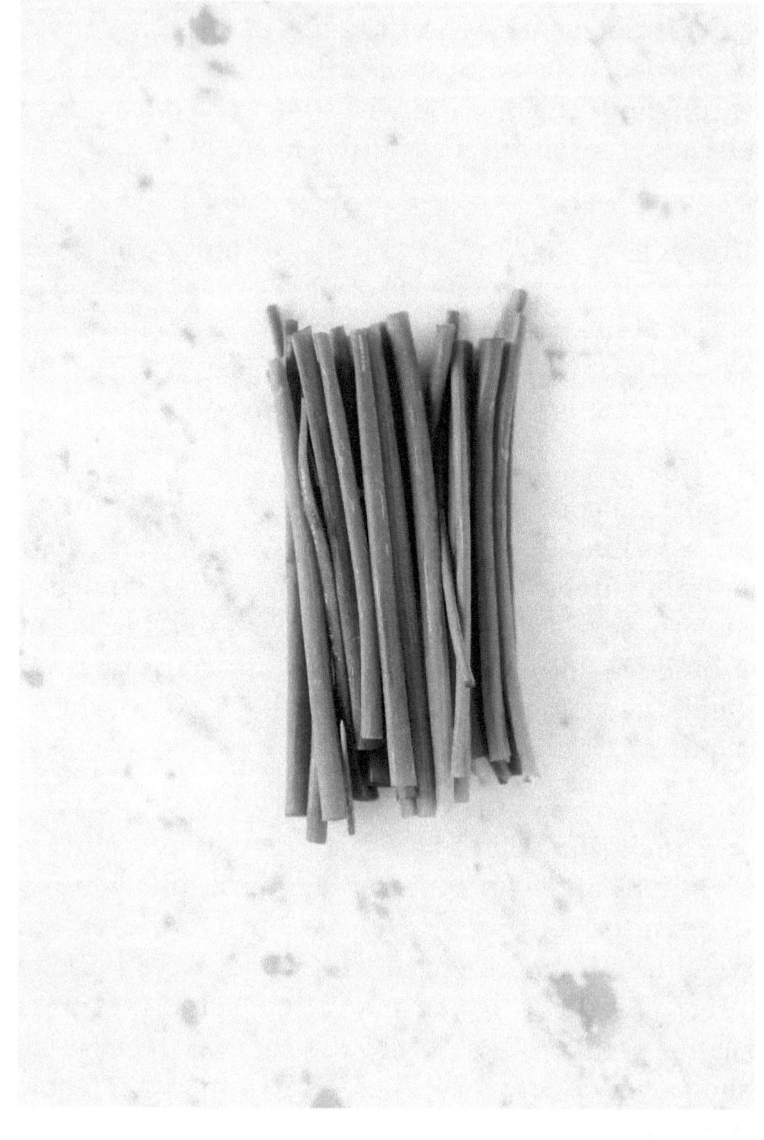

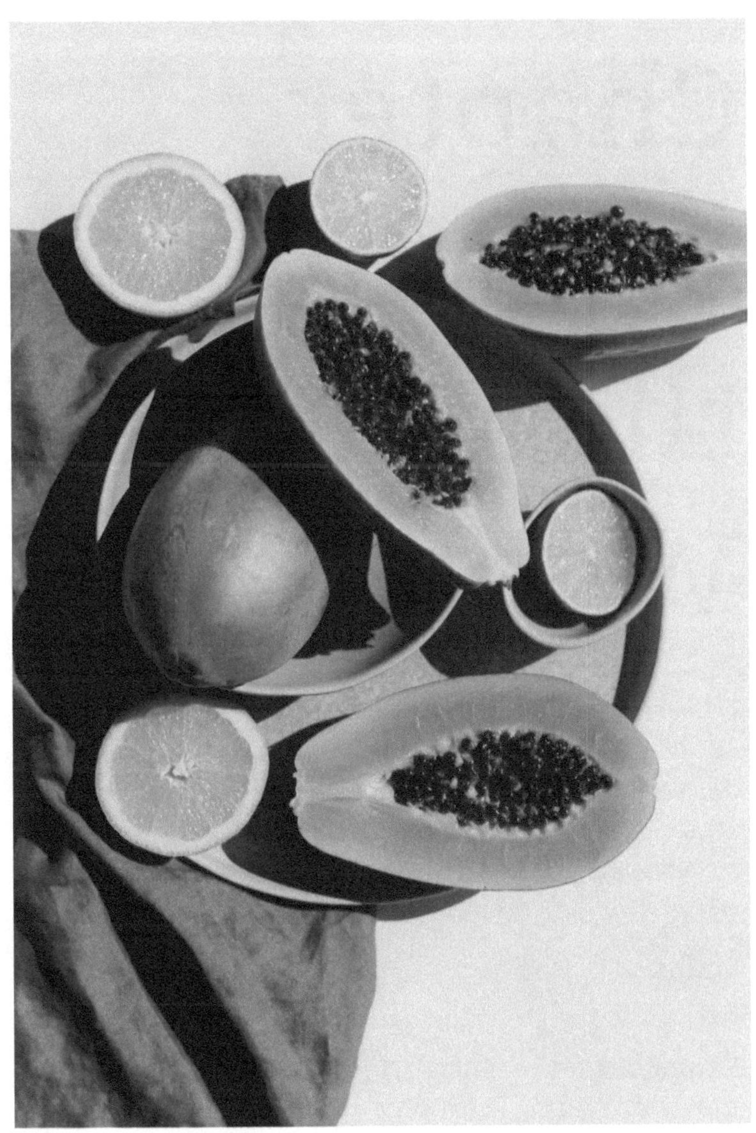

Chapter 3: Making the Most of Whole Foods

When transitioning to a vegan or plant-based diet, it can be helpful to learn how to cook with whole foods such as grains, legumes, and vegetables. Not only are these ingredients nutrient-dense, but they can also be versatile and delicious when prepared correctly.

Grains

Grains are an essential component of many vegan diets, providing carbohydrates and fiber. Whole grains, in particular, are packed with nutrients and are less processed than their refined counterparts. Brown rice, quinoa, bulgur, barley, and farro are all examples of whole grains that can be incorporated into your meals.

Cooking grains can seem intimidating, but with a little practice, it can become a breeze. One of the most important things to remember is to rinse the grains thoroughly before cooking to remove any debris or impurities. This step will also help to prevent the grains from becoming too sticky.

The ratio of water to grain can vary depending on the type of grain you are using, so it's important to follow the instructions on the package. Generally, a good rule of thumb is to use two cups of water for every cup of grain. After bringing the water to a boil, reduce the heat, cover the pot, and let the grains simmer until they are tender and the water has been absorbed. Fluff the grains with a fork and let them sit for a few minutes before serving.

Legumes

Legumes, such as lentils, chickpeas, and beans, are excellent sources of protein, fiber, and carbohydrates. They are also incredibly versatile, and can be used in a wide variety of dishes, from soups and stews to salads and spreads.

Cooking legumes from scratch can be time-consuming, but it's worth the effort. Soaking the legumes overnight can help to reduce cooking time and improve their texture. After soaking, rinse the legumes and transfer them to a pot with enough water to cover them by a few inches. Bring the water to a boil, reduce the heat, and let the legumes simmer until they are tender. Be sure to add salt towards the end of cooking, as adding it too early can toughen the legumes.

Canned legumes are also a convenient option, but be sure to rinse them thoroughly before using them to reduce the amount of sodium and other additives.

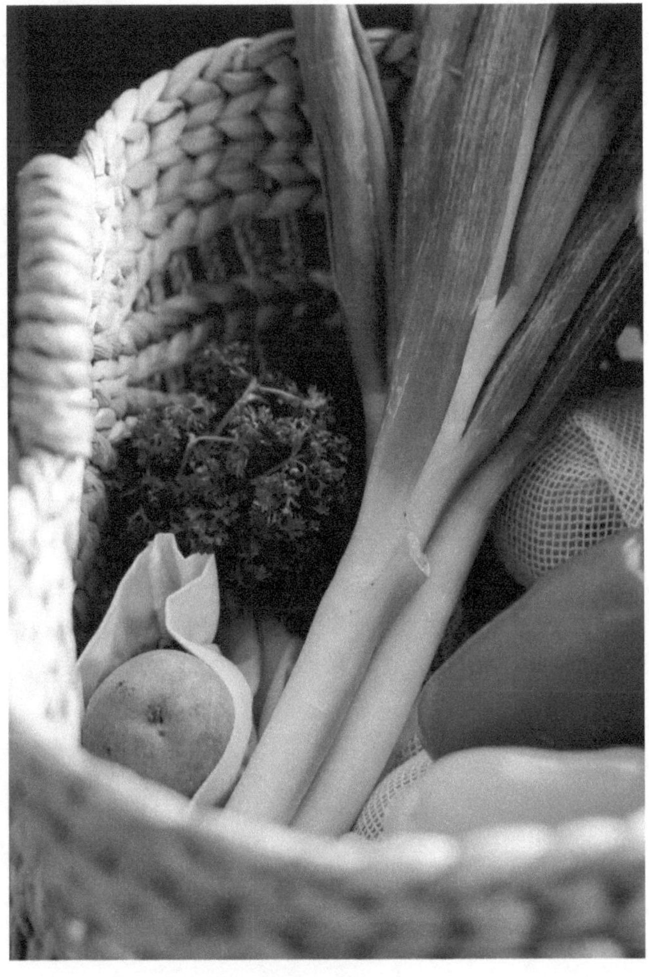

Vegetables

Vegetables are a key component of any healthy vegan diet. Incorporating a variety of colorful vegetables into your meals can help to ensure that you are getting a wide range of vitamins and minerals. Vegetables can be cooked in a variety of ways, including roasting, grilling, sautéing, and steaming.

One of the most important things to remember when cooking vegetables is to avoid overcooking them. This can cause them to become mushy and lose their flavor and nutrients. A good rule of thumb is to cook vegetables until they are tender but still have a slight crunch.

Roasting vegetables is a popular method, as it can help to bring out their natural sweetness and create a crispy texture. Simply toss your vegetables in a bit of oil and seasoning, and roast them in the oven at 400°F until they are tender and golden brown.

Steaming is another healthy and easy cooking method. Simply bring a pot of water to a boil, place your vegetables in a steamer basket, and steam until they are tender.

Incorporating whole foods into your vegan cooking can help to ensure that you are getting all of the nutrients you need to thrive. Experiment with different grains, legumes, and vegetables

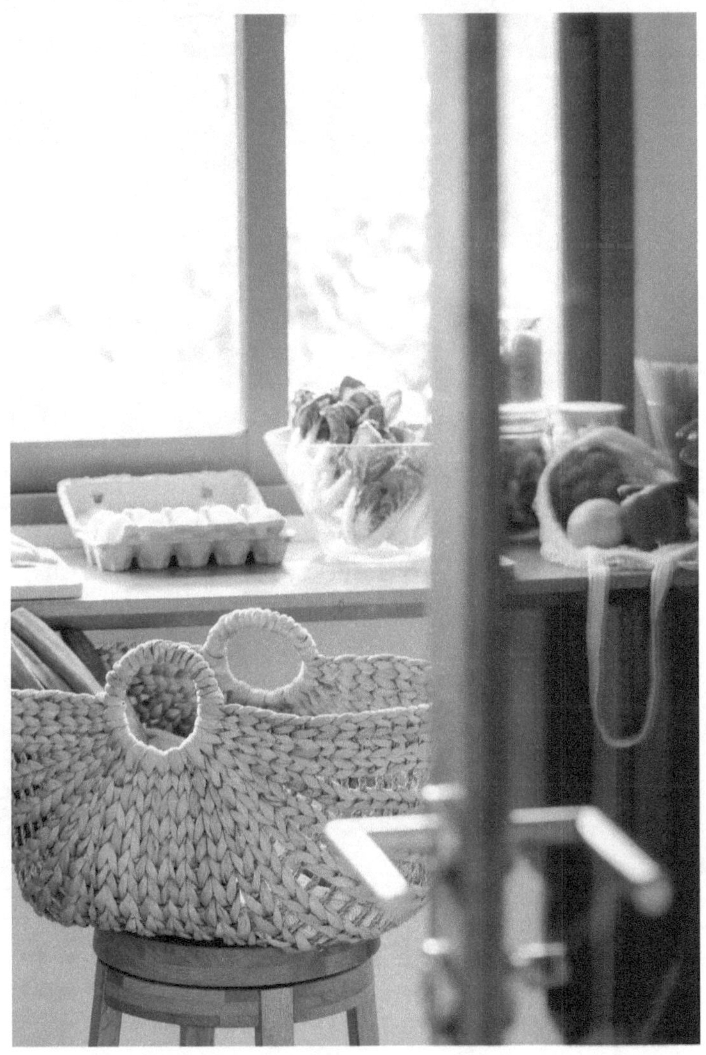

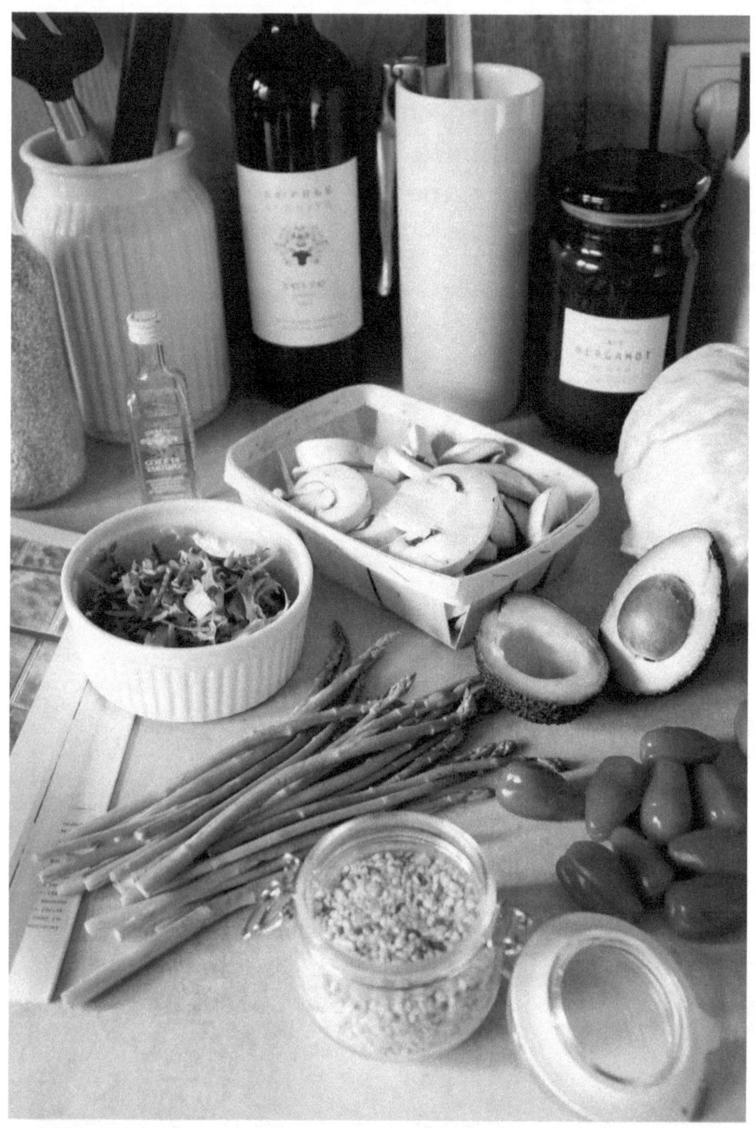

Chapter 4: Healthy Fats

and Oils: Navigating Vegan Cooking Oils and Incorporating Healthy Fats into Your Diet

When it comes to vegan and plant-based cooking, it's important to pay attention to the type of fats and oils that you use. Not all fats and oils are created equal, and some can be harmful to your health if consumed in excess. In this chapter, we'll explore some of the healthy fats and oils that you can incorporate into your diet, and provide tips on how to use them in your cooking.

First, it's important to understand the difference between fats and oils. Fats are solid at room temperature, while oils are liquid. Some examples of plant-based fats include coconut oil, cocoa butter, and avocado, while plant-based oils include olive oil, sesame oil, and sunflower oil. Both fats and oils provide the body with energy and are essential for the absorption of certain vitamins and minerals, such as vitamin A and vitamin E.

One of the most important considerations when it comes to healthy fats and oils is the type of fat that they contain. There are three main types of fats: saturated fats, monounsaturated fats, and polyunsaturated fats. Saturated fats, which are found in animal products such as butter and cheese, are considered to be the least healthy type of fat, as they can increase cholesterol levels and contribute to heart disease. Monounsaturated and polyunsaturated fats, on the other hand, are considered to be much healthier, and can even help to reduce the risk of heart disease.

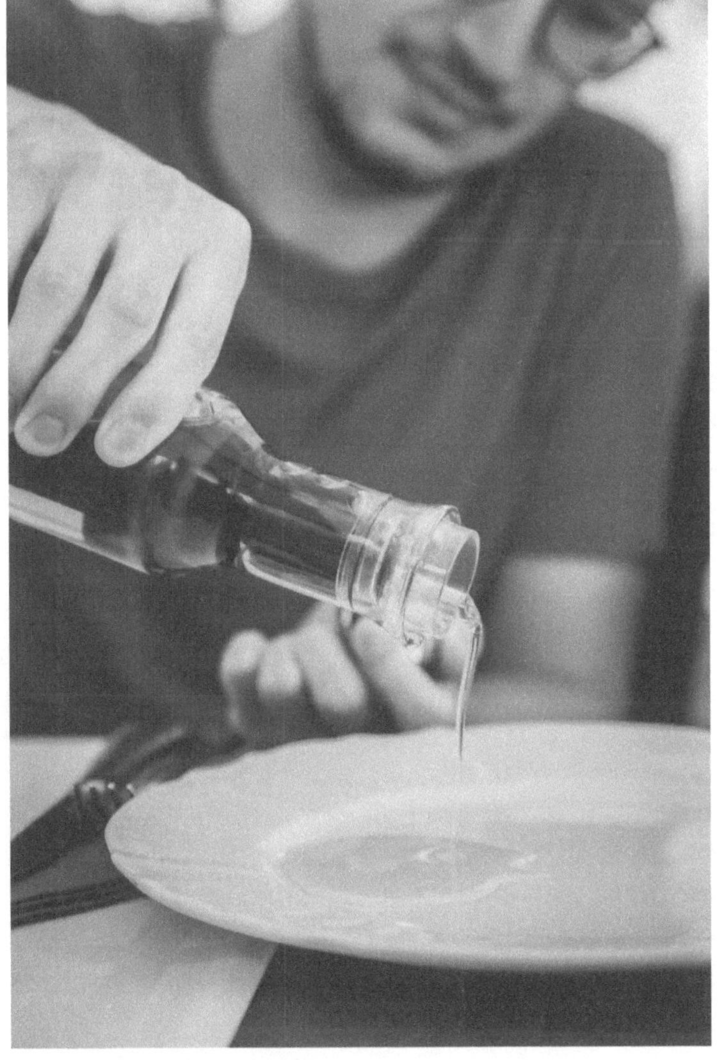

One of the healthiest oils for cooking is olive oil. Olive oil is rich in monounsaturated fats, which have been shown to improve cholesterol levels and reduce the risk of heart disease. Olive oil is also high in antioxidants, which can help to reduce inflammation in the body. When cooking with olive oil, it's important to choose a high-quality, extra-virgin variety, which has not been heavily processed.

Another healthy oil for cooking is coconut oil. Coconut oil is a saturated fat, but it contains medium-chain triglycerides (MCTs), which are metabolized differently than other types of fats. MCTs are quickly absorbed by the body and can be used for energy, making coconut oil a good choice for athletes and people who are trying to lose weight. Coconut oil also has antimicrobial properties, which can help to fight off infections.

Other healthy oils that you can use for cooking include avocado oil, which is rich in monounsaturated fats and has a high smoke point, making it a good choice for high-heat cooking methods such as frying and roasting. Sesame oil is another healthy oil that is rich in polyunsaturated fats and has a distinct nutty flavor that works well in Asian-style dishes.

When it comes to incorporating healthy fats into your diet, it's important to focus on whole foods rather than processed foods. Whole foods such as nuts, seeds, and avocado are rich in healthy fats, and can be easily incorporated into meals and snacks. Some good examples include adding avocado to your morning toast, sprinkling nuts and seeds on your salad, or using tahini (which is made from ground sesame seeds) in your salad dressings or dips.

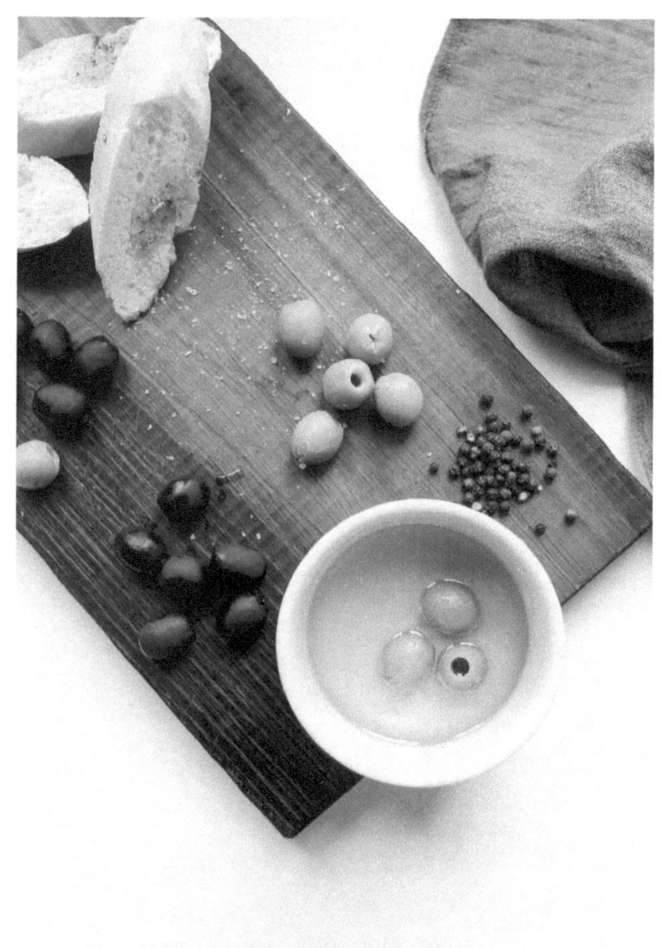

Another way to incorporate healthy fats into your diet is to choose plant-based milk and dairy alternatives. Many dairy alternatives, such as almond milk and coconut yogurt, are rich in healthy fats and can be used in place of dairy products in your cooking and baking.

In summary, when it comes to vegan and plant-based cooking, it's important to pay attention to the types of fats and oils that you use. Opt for healthy fats such as monounsaturated and polyunsaturated fats, and choose oils such as olive oil, coconut oil, and sesame oil.

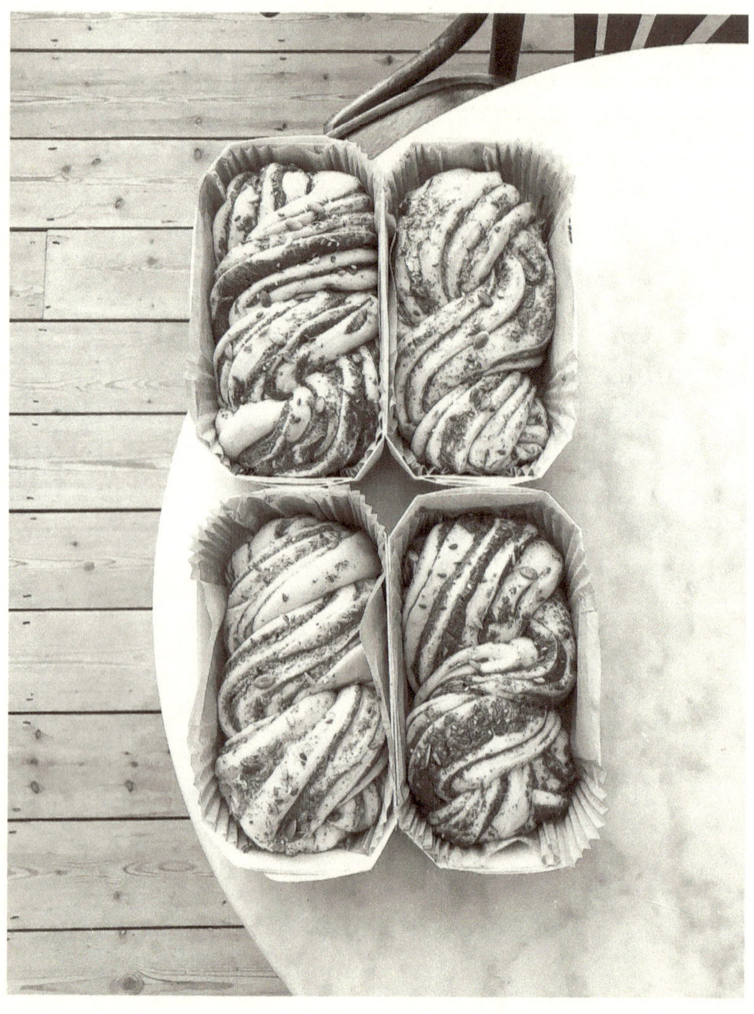

CHAPTER 5:
VEGAN BAKING

Baking can be a challenging aspect of vegan cooking. After all, many traditional baking recipes rely heavily on butter, eggs, and milk to achieve the desired texture and flavor. However, with a few simple substitutions and some practice, you can easily make vegan versions of your favorite baked goods that are just as delicious and satisfying as their non-vegan counterparts.

In this chapter, we'll explore some of the most important ingredients and techniques for successful vegan baking, as well as some of our favorite vegan baking recipes.

Key Ingredients for Vegan Baking

When it comes to vegan baking, there are a few key ingredients that you'll need to get comfortable with. These include:

Non-Dairy Milk: To replace cow's milk in recipes, you can use any non-dairy milk such as almond milk, soy milk, oat milk, or coconut milk. Be sure to use unsweetened varieties to avoid adding extra sweetness to your recipes.

Vegan Butter: Look for plant-based margarines or vegan butter alternatives, which can be found in most supermarkets these days. They can be used in equal amounts as traditional butter.

Aquafaba: Aquafaba is the liquid that comes from a can of chickpeas or other legumes. It can be whipped to create a meringue-like texture, which can be used as an egg white substitute in many recipes.

Flax and Chia Seeds: These can be used as an egg substitute by mixing them with water to form a gel-like consistency.

Vegan Yogurt or Silken Tofu: These can be used to replace eggs in baking and can add moisture and creaminess to your recipes.

Baking Techniques for Vegan Baking

When it comes to baking, there are a few key techniques that can help you achieve the best results. Here are some tips to keep in mind:

Measure Ingredients Accurately: Baking is a science, so it's important to measure your ingredients carefully. Use a kitchen scale to measure dry ingredients such as flour and sugar, and use measuring cups and spoons for liquids and other ingredients.

Don't Overmix: When mixing your ingredients, be careful not to overmix, as this can result in tough, dry baked goods. Mix until just combined and then stop.

Use the Right Pan: The type of pan you use can make a big difference in your baking. Non-stick metal pans are a good choice for most baked goods, while glass or ceramic pans may require a lower temperature and longer cooking time.

Check for Doneness: Use a toothpick or cake tester to check for doneness. If it comes out clean, your baked goods are ready. If not, bake for a few more minutes and check again.

Vegan Baking Recipes

Now that you're familiar with some of the key ingredients and techniques for vegan baking, it's time to get baking! Here are a few of our favorite vegan baking recipes:

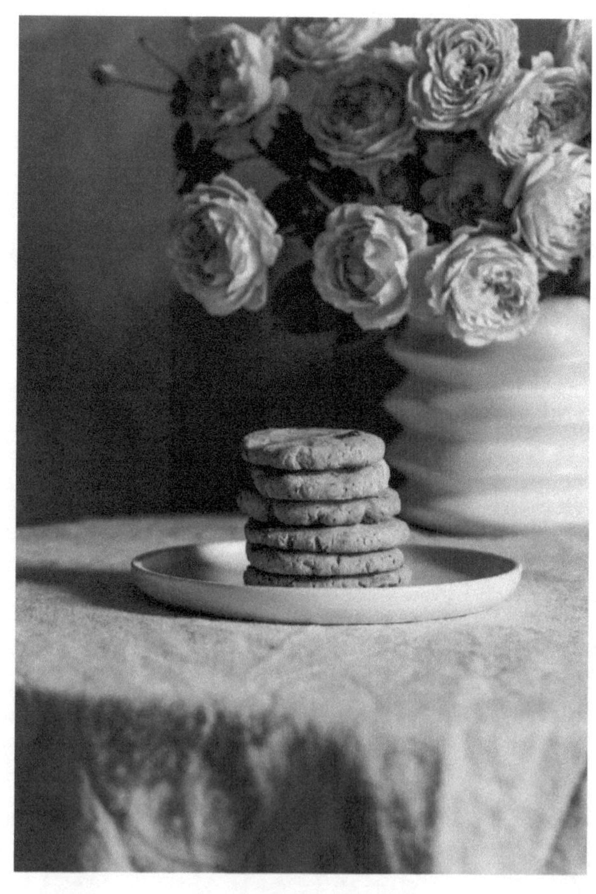

Vegan Chocolate Chip Cookies: Use vegan butter and flaxseeds instead of eggs to make a delicious and chewy batch of vegan chocolate chip cookies. These are perfect for an afternoon treat or dessert after dinner.

Vegan Banana Bread: This classic recipe is easy to make vegan with the help of some mashed ripe bananas and non-dairy milk. Add in some chopped walnuts or chocolate chips for extra flavor and texture.

Vegan Blueberry Muffins: These moist and fluffy muffins are a great option for breakfast or a snack. Use non-dairy milk and vegan yogurt to achieve a tender and light texture.

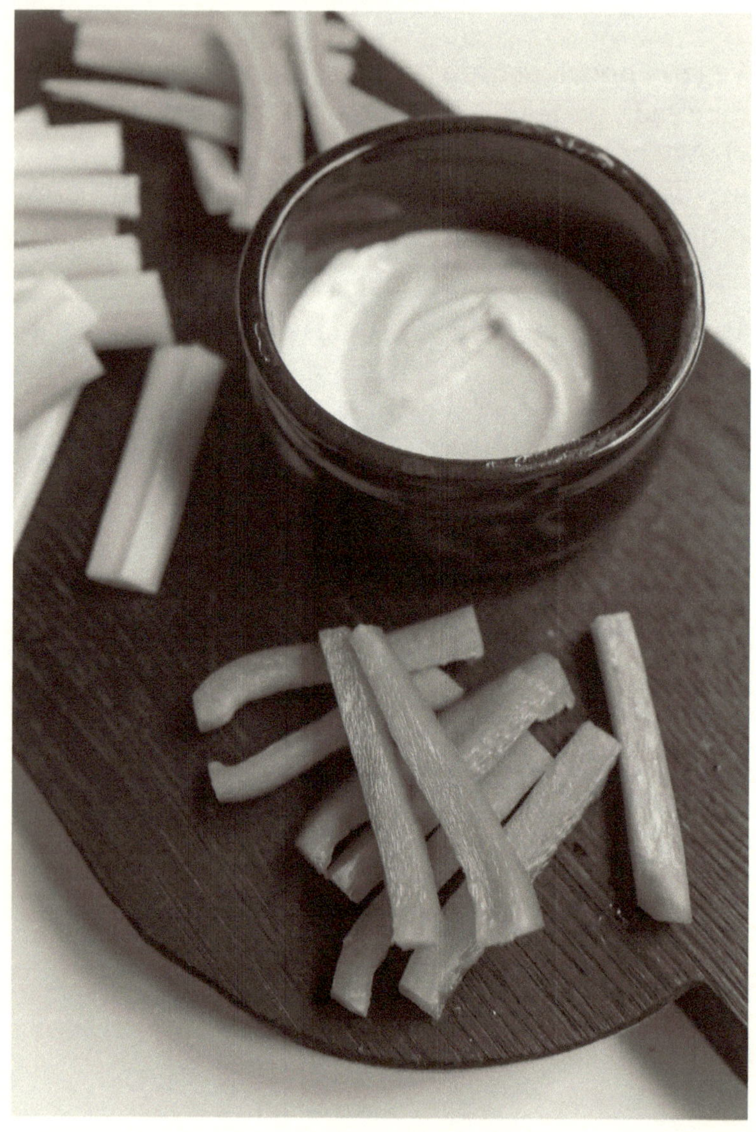

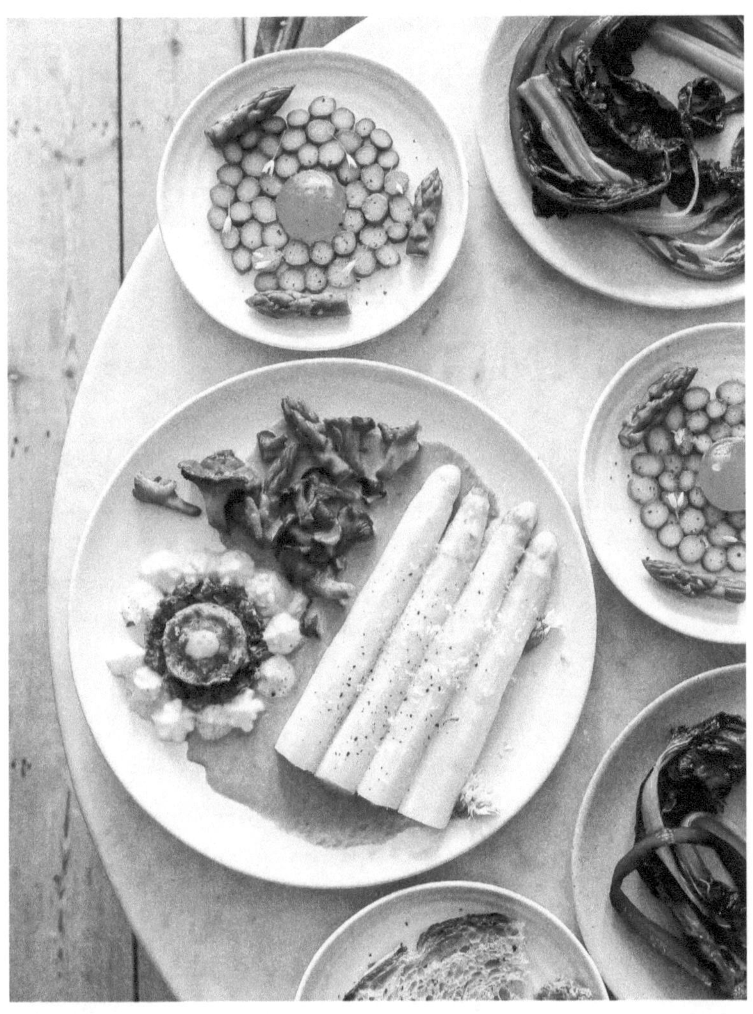

CHAPTER 6: SAUCES, DRESSINGS, AND CONDIMENTS

Sauces, dressings, and condiments are the finishing touches that can take a dish from good to great. They add flavor, texture, and sometimes a pop of color to any meal. In this chapter, we'll explore some delicious and healthy options for vegan and plant-based cooking.

Classic Sauces: Tomato, Marinara, and More

Tomato sauce is a classic choice for many pasta dishes, and it's simple to make. Start with canned or fresh tomatoes, and sauté onions and garlic until they're translucent. Add the tomatoes and some salt and pepper, and let the sauce simmer for 20-30 minutes. Other classic sauces include marinara, Alfredo, and pesto.

Creamy Dressings: Ranch, Caesar, and More

Ranch and Caesar dressings are creamy and

delicious, but most store-bought versions contain dairy. Luckily, it's easy to make a vegan version at home. For ranch dressing, blend together vegan mayonnaise, non-dairy milk, and spices like dill and garlic. For Caesar dressing, use a base of cashews or silken tofu, and add nutritional yeast, lemon juice, and garlic for flavor.

Spicy Condiments: Sriracha, Harissa, and More

If you love a little heat in your food, there are plenty of spicy condiments to choose from. Sriracha is a popular choice for adding spice to any dish, from noodles to tofu. Harissa, a North African chili paste, is another flavorful option. Mix it with some tahini and lemon juice for a tasty sauce.

Nut-Based Sauces: Peanut, Cashew, and More

Peanut sauce is a staple in many Asian cuisines, and it's easy to make a vegan version. Just blend together peanut butter, soy sauce, lime juice, and some hot sauce if you like it spicy. Cashew sauce is another nut-based option that's creamy and versatile. Blend together soaked cashews, water, lemon juice, and spices for a flavorful sauce.

Vinaigrettes: Balsamic, Lemon, and More

Vinaigrettes are light and tangy, and they're perfect for dressing salads or roasted vegetables. Balsamic vinaigrette is a classic, and it's easy to make at home with balsamic vinegar, olive oil, and some Dijon mustard. Lemon vinaigrette is another simple option that's refreshing and bright. Mix together lemon juice, olive oil, and some garlic and honey for a flavorful dressing.

Sweet Sauces: Caramel, Chocolate, and More

Dessert sauces can be just as delicious as savory ones, and they're easy to make without dairy. Caramel sauce can be made with coconut cream and sugar, and it's perfect for drizzling over ice cream or cakes. Chocolate sauce is another sweet option, and it's easy to make with cocoa powder, coconut oil, and a sweetener like maple syrup.

Chutneys and Salsas: Mango, Tomato, and More

Chutneys and salsas are flavorful and versatile, and they can be used as a dip or a topping. Mango chutney is a sweet and tangy option that's great with Indian food, and it's easy to make with diced mango, vinegar, and spices. Tomato salsa is a classic that's perfect for dipping tortilla chips or topping tacos. Mix together diced tomatoes, onion, cilantro, and lime juice for a fresh and tasty salsa.

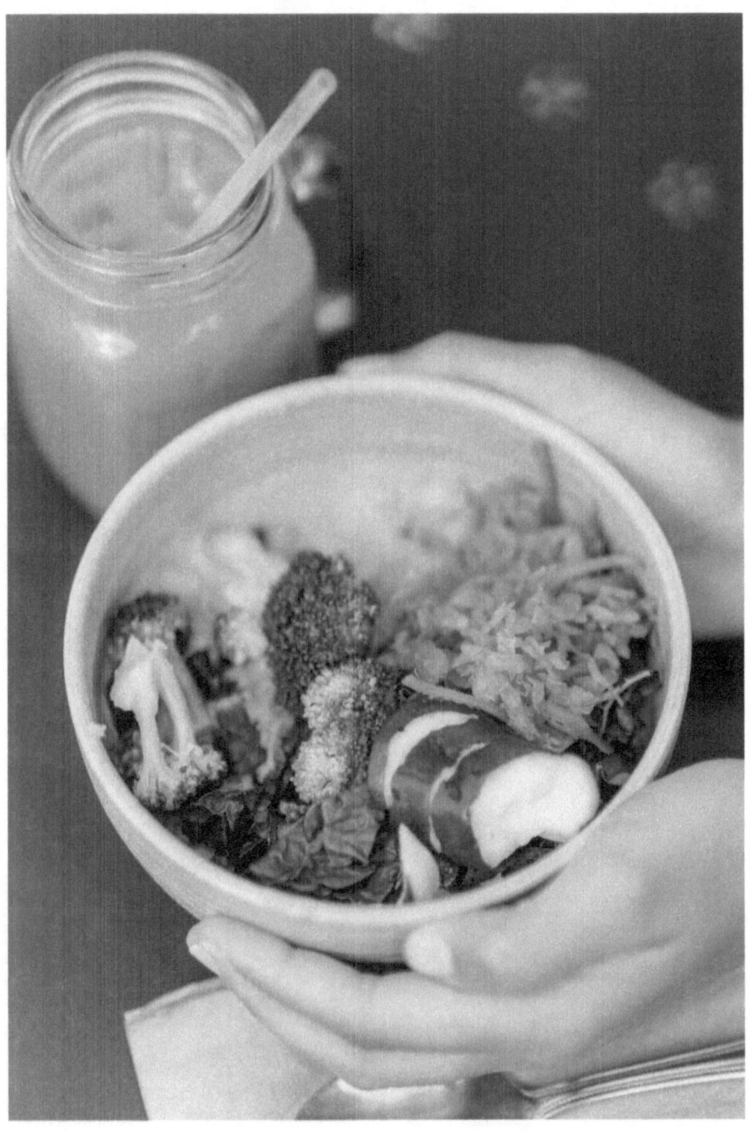

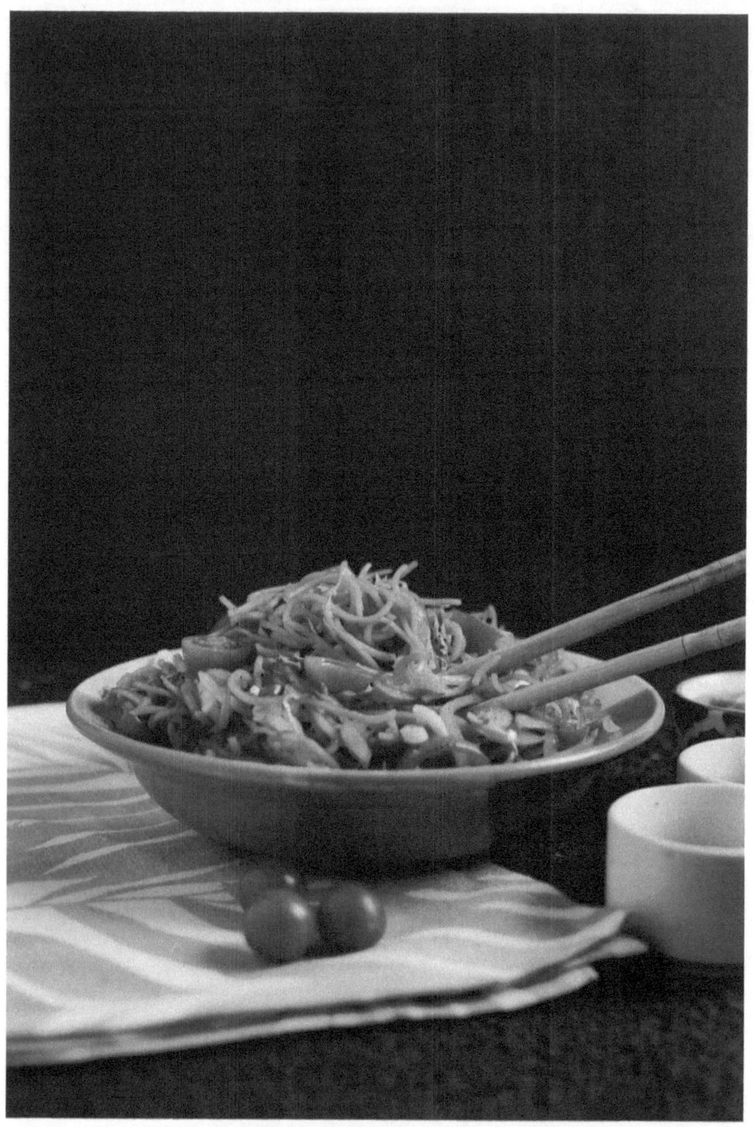

Chapter 7: International

Vegan Cuisine - Exploring the Best Plant-Based Recipes from Around the World

One of the most exciting aspects of vegan cooking is the diversity of cuisines and cultures that you can explore. From the hearty stews of Eastern Europe to the fragrant curries of Southeast Asia, there are endless possibilities when it comes to plant-based cooking from around the world. In this chapter, we'll explore some of the best vegan recipes and cooking styles from different regions of the globe.

Let's start with the Mediterranean. The cuisine of this region is characterized by fresh, vibrant ingredients like tomatoes, olives, and herbs, and is a great place to start if you're new to vegan cooking. One popular Mediterranean dish is tabbouleh, a refreshing salad made with bulgur wheat, tomatoes, cucumbers, and lots of parsley and mint. Another classic is hummus, a creamy dip made from chickpeas, tahini, and lemon juice. Both of these dishes are easy to make and are perfect for a light lunch or snack.

Moving on to Asia, there are countless vegan options to explore. In Japan, for example, you can try your hand at making sushi rolls filled with avocado, cucumber, and pickled vegetables. In India, you can experiment with making your own chana masala, a spicy and savory chickpea curry that is perfect served over rice or with naan bread. And in Thailand, you can create a vibrant green papaya salad with a dressing made from lime juice, fish sauce (use vegan alternative), and chili.

If you're looking for something heartier, then the stews and casseroles of Eastern Europe are a great place to start. A hearty bean and vegetable goulash is a popular dish in Hungary, while a filling cabbage roll stuffed with grains and mushrooms is a classic in Poland. These dishes are perfect for cold winter days and can easily be made in large batches for meal prep.

Moving on to South America, there are many vegan dishes that are both delicious and nutritious. A classic Brazilian dish is feijoada, a hearty black bean stew that is typically served with rice and farofa, a toasted cassava flour mixture. In Peru, you can try making a flavorful quinoa and vegetable stir-fry, while in Mexico, you can create your own vegan tacos filled with roasted sweet potato and black beans.

Finally, let's not forget about the Middle East. This region is known for its use of spices and herbs, and there are many vegan dishes to explore here. One of the most popular is falafel, which is made from ground chickpeas, herbs, and spices and then fried until crispy. Another great Middle Eastern dish is muhammara, a dip made from roasted red peppers, walnuts, and breadcrumbs that is perfect served with pita bread.

The great thing about vegan cuisine is that it's not only delicious but also healthy and sustainable. By exploring different cooking styles and ingredients from around the world, you can broaden your culinary horizons while also supporting a plant-based lifestyle that is good for your body and the planet. So whether you're craving something spicy, sweet, or savory, there's a vegan dish out there that will satisfy your taste buds and nourish your body.

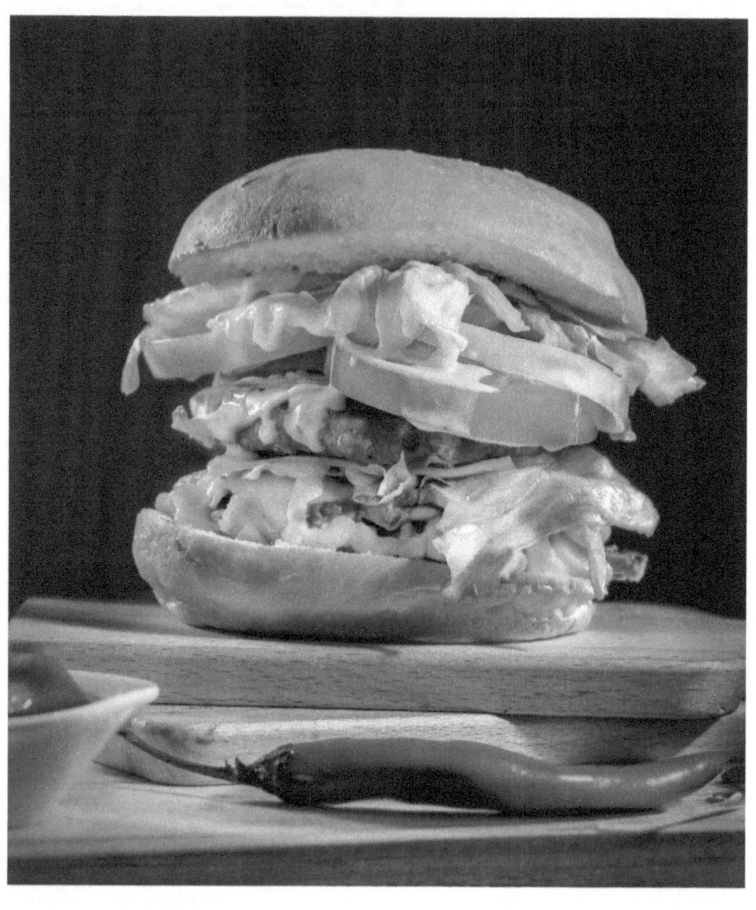

CHAPTER 8: VEGAN COMFORT FOOD: SATISFYING YOUR CRAVINGS FOR BURGERS, FRIES, AND MAC & CHEESE, THE VEGAN WAY

When transitioning to a vegan or plant-based diet, it's natural to miss some of your favorite comfort foods. But fear not, because with a little creativity and some key ingredients, you can enjoy all the familiar tastes and textures without the animal products. In this chapter, we'll explore some classic comfort foods and how to make them vegan-friendly.

Burgers: Perhaps one of the most beloved comfort foods, the classic burger can easily be made vegan. You can use store-bought vegan burger patties or make your own using black beans, lentils, mushrooms, or tofu as a base. Top your burger with all your favorite fixings, such as lettuce, tomato, onion, pickles, and vegan cheese. You can also make your own special sauce using vegan mayo, ketchup, mustard, and relish.

Fries: French fries are a staple side dish for burgers, but they're also delicious on their own. To make them vegan, simply cut potatoes into strips and fry them in a neutral oil such as vegetable or canola oil. For added flavor, you can sprinkle them with salt and pepper or season them with garlic powder, paprika, or chili flakes. For a healthier alternative, you can also bake your fries in the oven.

Mac & Cheese: Creamy, cheesy, and comforting, mac & cheese is a childhood favorite for many. To make a vegan version, you can use plant-based milk such as almond or soy milk, and vegan cheese such as Daiya or Follow Your Heart. You can also add nutritional yeast for a cheesy flavor and cashews for creaminess. For a healthier option, you can use whole wheat or gluten-free pasta and add veggies such as broccoli, peas, or spinach.

Pizza: Who doesn't love pizza? Luckily, it's easy to make a vegan version at home or order one at a vegan-friendly restaurant. You can use a pre-made pizza crust or make your own using flour, yeast, and water. For the sauce, use a tomato-based sauce or make your own using crushed tomatoes and Italian herbs. Top your pizza with vegan cheese, veggies such as mushrooms, onions, and peppers, and vegan pepperoni or sausage.

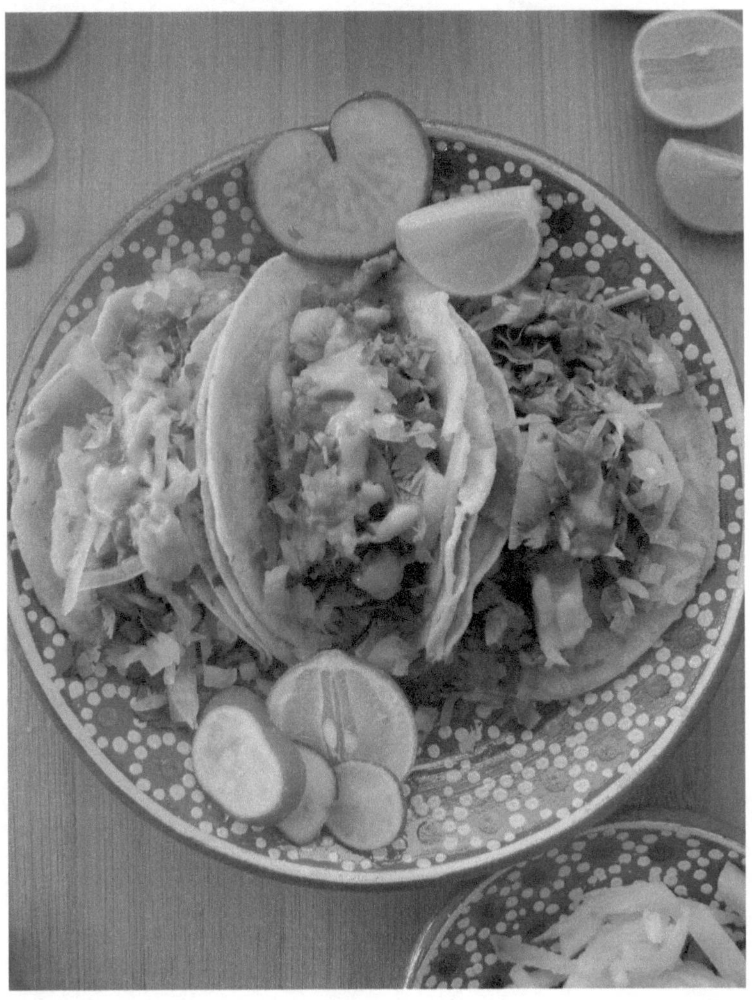

Tacos: Tacos are a fun and easy meal that can be easily made vegan. Use black or pinto beans, tempeh, or tofu as a protein source, and load up your tacos with all your favorite toppings such as avocado, salsa, lettuce, and vegan cheese. You can also make your own tortillas using masa harina and water, or use store-bought corn or flour tortillas.

Grilled Cheese: There's nothing quite like a grilled cheese sandwich for a quick and easy meal. To make a vegan version, use vegan bread such as sourdough or whole wheat, and vegan cheese such as Chao or Violife. You can also add tomato, avocado, or vegan bacon for extra flavor.

Chili: Chili is a hearty and comforting meal that's easy to make vegan. Use beans, lentils, or TVP (textured vegetable protein) as a protein source, and load up your chili with veggies such as onion, bell pepper, and tomato. For added flavor, you can use chili powder, cumin, and paprika. Serve your chili with vegan sour cream or avocado and vegan cornbread.

Mashed Potatoes: Creamy and comforting, mashed potatoes are a perfect side dish for any meal. To make them vegan, use vegan butter such as Earth Balance or Miyoko's, and plant-based milk such as almond or soy milk. You can also add garlic, chives, or vegan cheese

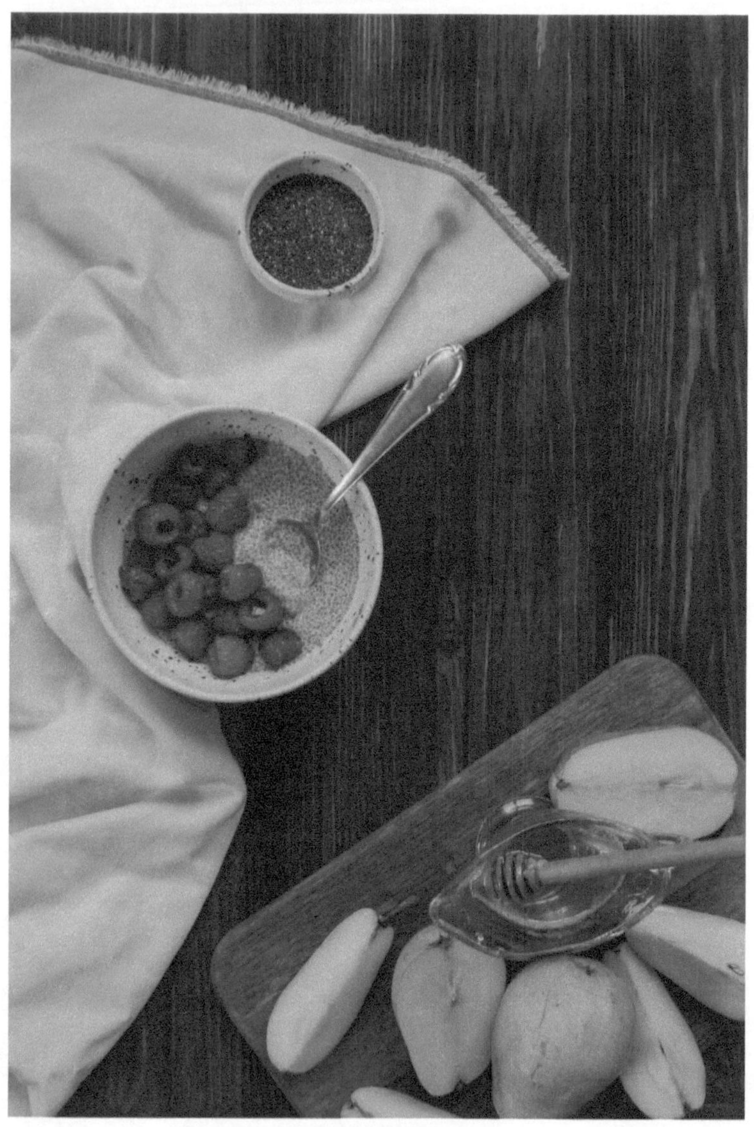

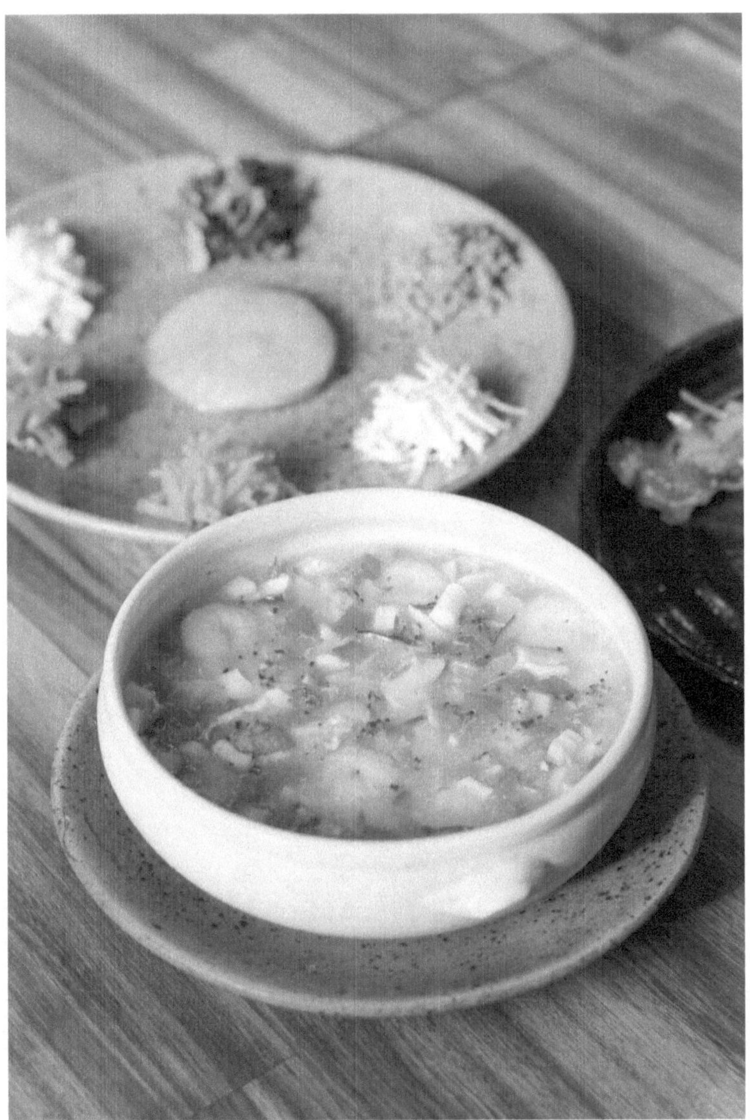

Chapter 9: Meal Planning

and Batch Cooking: Simplifying Your Vegan Cooking Routine for a Busy Lifestyle

As a busy person, you know how challenging it can be to eat healthy and flavorful meals while juggling a packed schedule. That's where meal planning and batch cooking come in. With a little bit of time and effort, you can create a week's worth of delicious and nutritious vegan meals that can be easily reheated and enjoyed throughout the week.

Meal Planning

The first step to meal planning is to set aside some time each week to sit down and plan out your meals. This can be as simple as making a list of the meals you want to eat for the week and then creating a shopping list for the ingredients you'll need. You can also create a more detailed plan that includes breakfast, lunch, dinner, and snacks for each day of the week.

When meal planning, it's important to consider your schedule and plan accordingly. If you know you'll be working late one night, for example, plan for a meal that can be easily reheated or made in advance. If you have a busy morning, consider making overnight oats or a breakfast casserole that can be easily heated up.

Batch Cooking

Batch cooking involves preparing large quantities of food at once, so you have meals ready to go throughout the week. This can be especially helpful if you have a busy schedule and don't have time to cook every day.

To get started with batch cooking, choose a few recipes that you enjoy and that can be easily reheated. This could be a vegan chili, a vegetable curry, or a quinoa salad. Make a big batch of the recipe and portion it out into individual containers. Store the containers in the fridge or freezer, and you'll have healthy meals ready to go throughout the week.

When batch cooking, it's important to have the right tools and equipment. A large pot or slow cooker can be great for making big batches of soup or chili. A baking sheet can be used to roast vegetables or make sheet pan meals. Glass containers with lids are ideal for storing your prepped meals in the fridge or freezer.

Tips for Success

Here are a few tips to help you succeed with meal planning and batch cooking:

Plan your meals around ingredients that are in season and on sale. This will help you save money and enjoy the best flavors.

Use the same ingredients in different ways throughout the week. For example, if you're roasting sweet potatoes for one meal, you can use the leftovers in a salad or as a side dish for another meal.

Don't be afraid to mix and match recipes. You can use the same base ingredients in different recipes to create variety throughout the week.

Consider prepping ingredients in advance. For example, you can chop vegetables or cook grains on the weekend, so they're ready to go when it's time to cook.

Use sauces and condiments to add flavor to your meals. A simple dressing or sauce can turn a basic meal into something delicious and satisfying.

Conclusion

Meal planning and batch cooking are great ways to simplify your vegan cooking routine and ensure that you have healthy meals ready to go throughout the week. By setting aside a little bit of time each week to plan and prep your meals, you can enjoy delicious and nutritious vegan food without the stress and hassle of daily cooking. With the right tools, ingredients, and tips, you'll be a meal planning and batch cooking pro in no time!

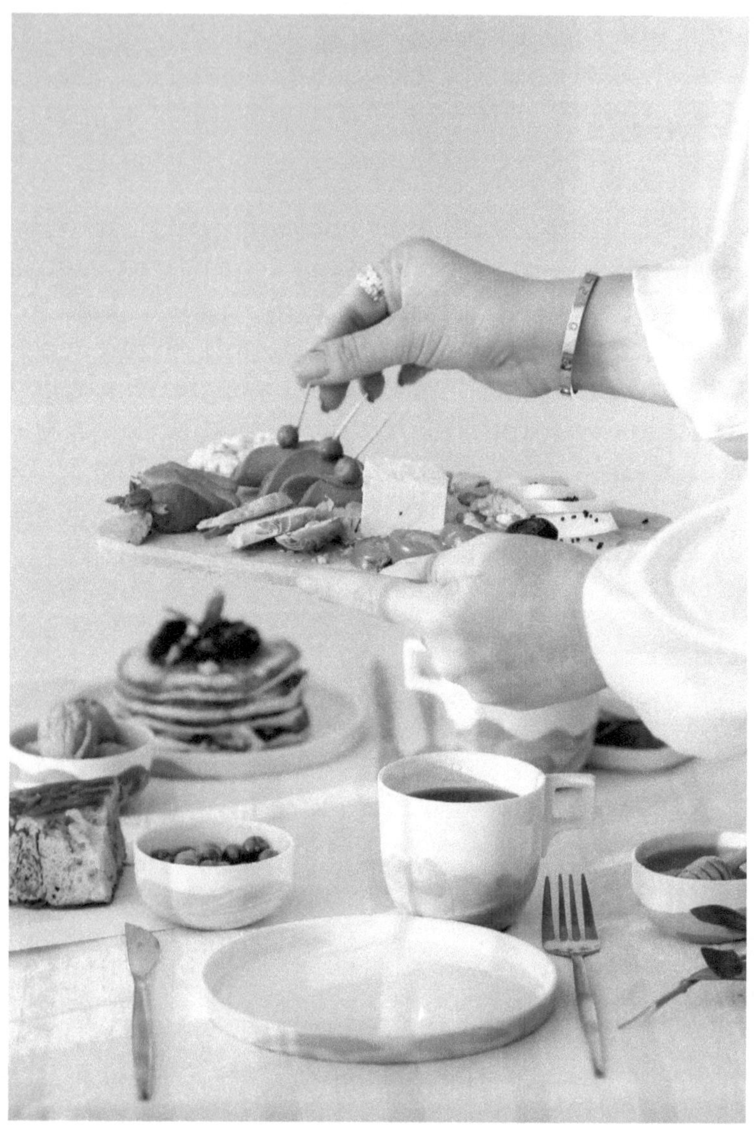

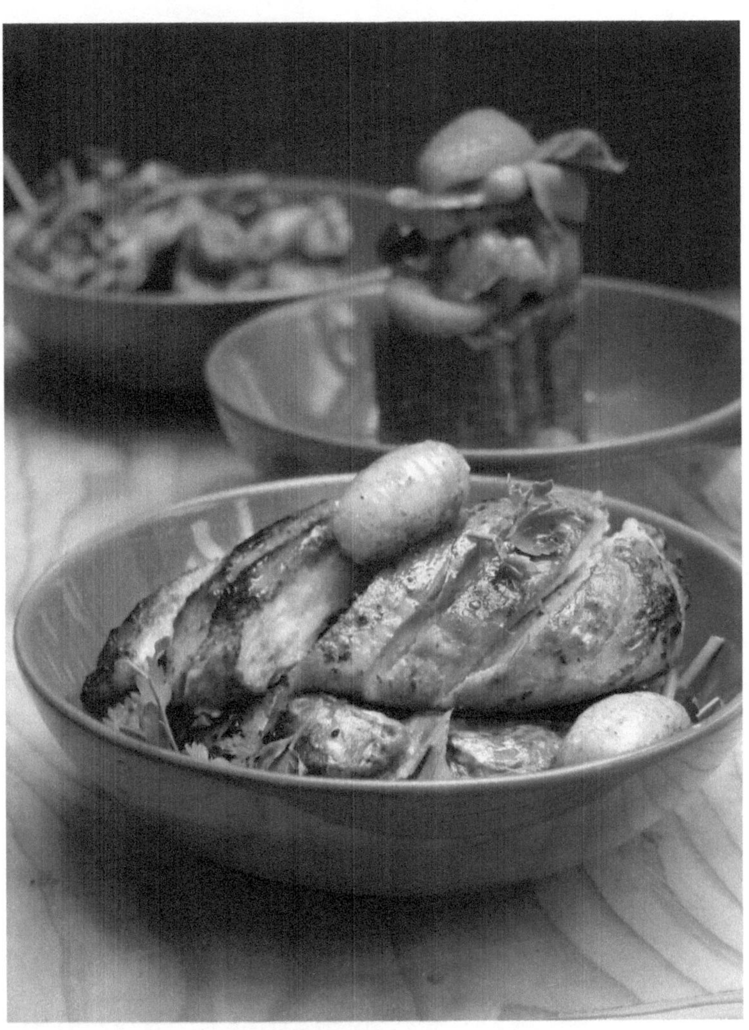

Chapter 10:

Hosting a Vegan Feast

As a vegan, hosting a gathering or dinner party can sometimes feel daunting. It can be difficult to plan and prepare a delicious menu that caters to all dietary needs, without compromising on taste and satisfaction. However, with a little bit of planning and creativity, hosting a vegan feast can be an enjoyable and rewarding experience.

In this chapter, we will provide you with some helpful tips and advice on how to plan and execute a vegan feast that will impress your guests.

Start with the Menu

The key to hosting a successful vegan feast is to plan your menu carefully. Begin by considering your guests' dietary requirements and preferences. Are any of your guests gluten-free, nut-free or have any other specific dietary restrictions? Make sure you accommodate these needs when planning your menu.

When it comes to the actual menu, consider serving a mix of dishes that are both savory and sweet. Offer a variety of appetizers, mains, sides, and desserts that will appeal to a range of tastes.

Get Creative with Your Ingredients

Don't be afraid to get creative with your ingredients when planning your menu. Vegan cooking offers a wide range of delicious and healthy ingredients that can be used to create impressive dishes. Experiment with different spices, herbs, and sauces to add flavor and depth to your dishes.

Try to incorporate some plant-based protein sources such as legumes, tofu, tempeh, or seitan into your menu. These ingredients are versatile and can be used in a variety of dishes such as salads, curries, stir-fries, or burgers.

Timing is Key

Timing is crucial when hosting a dinner party or gathering. Plan your menu in a way that allows you to spend as much time as possible with your guests. Prepare dishes ahead of time and choose dishes that can be served at room temperature, such as salads or dips. This will help you to be able to focus on socializing and enjoying your guests' company.

Presentation Matters

Just because you're serving a vegan meal, it doesn't mean it has to be boring or lackluster. Make sure you take the time to present your dishes in an attractive and appealing manner. Use colorful vegetables, herbs, and fruits to add some visual interest to your plates. Garnish your dishes with nuts, seeds, or edible flowers for an extra touch of elegance.

Have Fun with Desserts

Desserts are a great way to impress your guests and show them that vegan food can be both delicious and indulgent. Experiment with different vegan ingredients such as coconut cream, aquafaba, or vegan chocolate to make decadent desserts such as cakes, pies, or ice cream.

Remember, It's Not About Perfection

Hosting a vegan feast can be a bit overwhelming, especially if you're new to vegan cooking. However, it's important to remember that your guests are there to enjoy your company and the overall experience, not to critique your cooking skills. Don't be too hard on yourself if something doesn't go according to plan. The most important thing is to enjoy the moment and have fun with your guests.

Hosting a vegan feast can be a fun and rewarding experience. With a bit of planning and creativity, you can create a delicious and satisfying meal that will impress your guests. Remember to consider your guests' dietary requirements and preferences, get creative with your ingredients, and have fun with your desserts. With these tips in mind, you'll be well on your way to hosting a successful and enjoyable vegan feast.

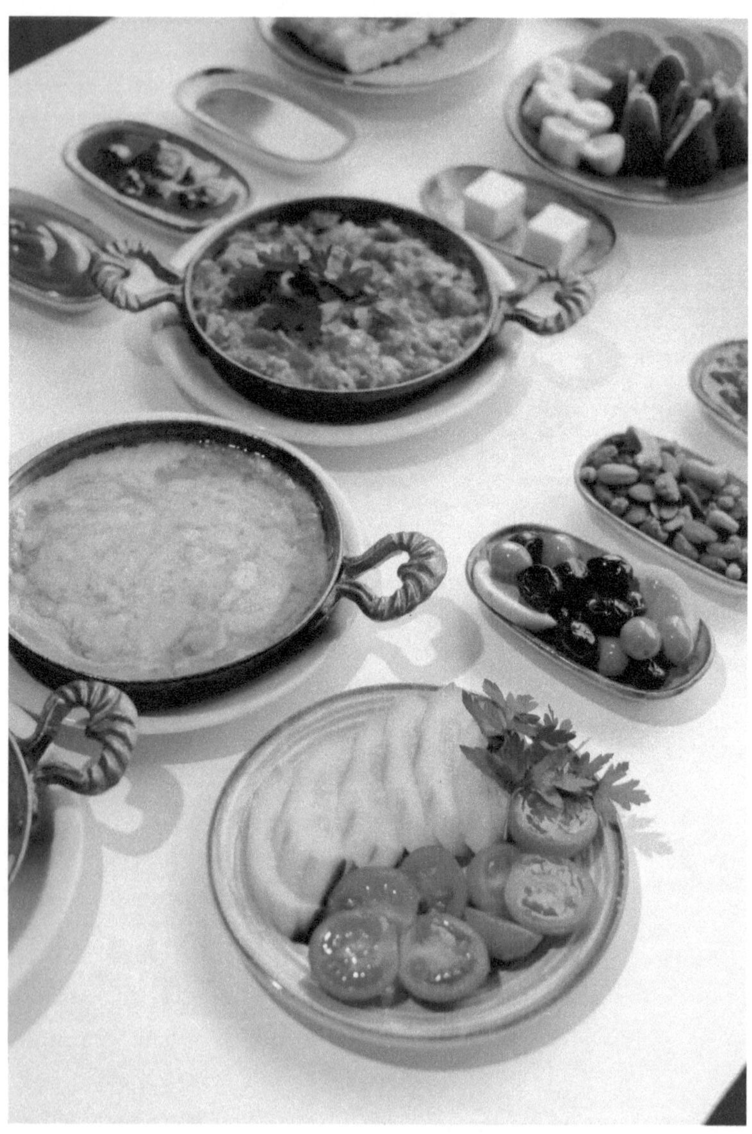

As we come to the end of this book on vegan and plant-based cooking, we hope that you've gained a deeper appreciation for the incredible flavors, health benefits, and ethical considerations that come with choosing a plant-based lifestyle. Whether you're a longtime vegan, a curious omnivore, or someone just starting to explore the world of vegan cooking, we believe that this book has something to offer you.

One of the most important things to keep in mind when it comes to vegan and plant-based cooking is that it's not an all-or-nothing proposition. You don't have to be 100% vegan all the time to reap the benefits of this way of eating. Every little bit counts, and even small changes in your diet can have a big impact on your health, the environment, and animal welfare. Whether it's swapping out meat for beans in a chili recipe, adding a handful of leafy greens to your morning smoothie, or trying out a new vegan restaurant in your neighborhood, every step towards a plant-based lifestyle is a step in the right direction.

At the same time, we understand that making the switch to a vegan diet can be challenging, especially if you're used to eating a lot of animal products. It can be hard to know where to start, what to buy, and how to prepare tasty and satisfying meals without meat, dairy, and eggs. That's where this book comes in. We've tried to provide you with the information, recipes, and resources you need to get started with vegan cooking, whether you're a complete beginner or an experienced chef.

Of course, we recognize that there are many different reasons why people choose to eat a plant-based diet, and we've tried to address some of the most common concerns throughout this book. Whether you're motivated by health, environmental, or ethical concerns (or some combination of all three), there are compelling reasons to give veganism a try. And the good news is that you don't have to sacrifice flavor or variety in the process. With so many delicious and nutritious plant-based foods out there, there's truly something for everyone.

Finally, we want to emphasize that veganism is not just a diet, but a lifestyle. It's about living in a way that reflects your values and makes a positive impact on the world around you. That can mean choosing cruelty-free products, reducing your waste, supporting local and organic agriculture, and more. By embracing a plant-based lifestyle, you're not only doing something good for yourself, but for the planet and its inhabitants as well.